My Paleo Diet Recipe Book

Easy & Healthy Recipes to Make Unforgettable Dishes

Carol Galindo

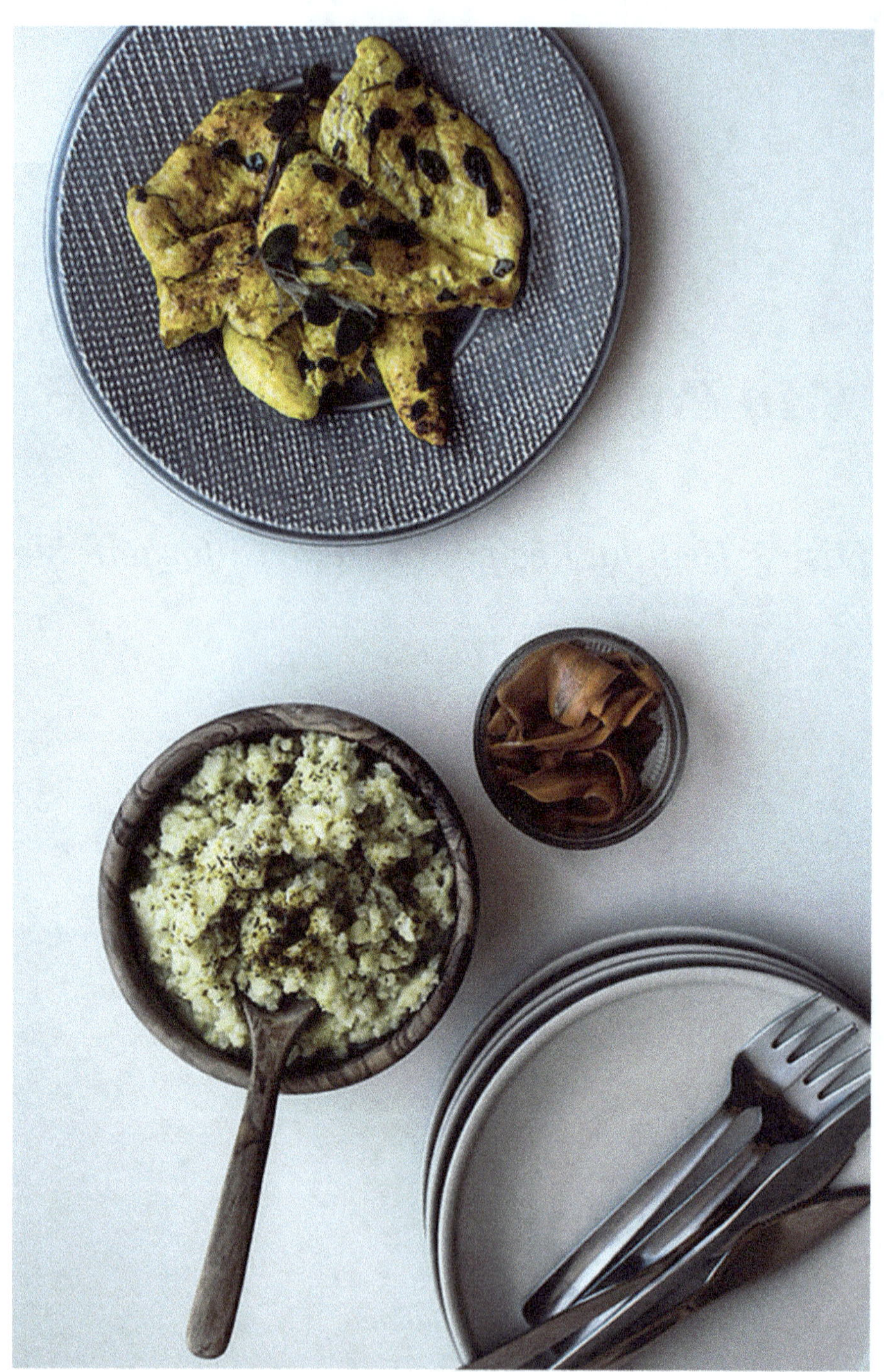

© Copyright 2021 - All rights reserved.

The content contained within this book may not be reproduced, duplicated or transmitted without direct written permission from the author or the publisher.

Under no circumstances will any blame or legal responsibility be held against the publisher, or author, for any damages, reparation, or monetary loss due to the information contained within this book. Either directly or indirectly.

Legal Notice:

This book is copyright protected. This book is only for personal use. You cannot amend, distribute, sell, use, quote or paraphrase any part, or the content within this book, without the consent of the author or publisher.

Disclaimer Notice:

Please note the information contained within this document is for educational and entertainment purposes only. All effort has been executed to present accurate, up to date, and reliable, complete information. No warranties of any kind are declared or implied. Readers acknowledge that the author is not engaging in the rendering of legal, financial, medical or professional advice. The content within this book has been derived from various sources. Please consult a licensed professional before attempting any techniques outlined in this book.

By reading this document, the reader agrees that under no circumstances is the author responsible for any losses, direct or indirect, which are incurred as a result of the use of information contained within this document, including, but not limited to, — errors, omissions, or inaccuracies.

Table of Contents

Paleo Seafood and Fish Recipes

Basil Scallops Mix

Servings: 2

Preparation time: 15 minutes

Cooking time: 0 minutes

Ingredients:

- 6 scallops, diced
- A pinch of sea salt
- Black pepper to taste
- 3 strawberries, chopped
- 1 tablespoon extra-virgin olive oil
- 1 tablespoon green onions, minced
- Juice from ½ lemon

* ½ tablespoon basil leaves, finely chopped

Directions:

1. In a bowl, mix all the ingredients, toss and keep in the fridge for 15 minutes.

2. Keep the tartar in the fridge until ready to serve.

Nutritional value/serving: calories 149, fat 7,8, carbs 4,8, fiber 0,5, protein 15,3

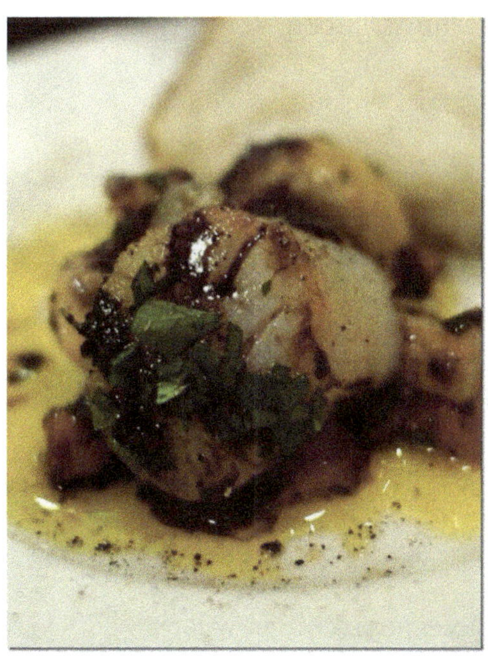

Creole Shrimp Mix

Servings: 4

Preparation time: 10 minutes

Cooking time: 10 minutes

Ingredients:

- ½ pound turkey meat, already cooked and sliced

- ½ pound shrimp, peeled and deveined

- 2 tablespoons extra virgin olive oil

- 2 zucchinis, cubed

- A pinch of sea salt

- Black pepper to taste

For the Creole seasoning:

- ½ tablespoon garlic powder

- 2 tablespoons paprika

- ½ tablespoon onion powder

- ¼ tablespoon oregano, dried

- ½ tablespoon chili powder

- ¼ tablespoon thyme, dried

Directions:

1. In a bowl, mix paprika with garlic powder, onion one, chili powder, oregano, and thyme and stir well.

2. In another bowl, mix shrimp with turkey meat, zucchini, and oil and toss to coat.

3. Pour paprika mix over shrimp mix and stir well.

4. Arrange turkey, shrimp, and zucchini on skewers alternating pieces, season with a pinch of sea salt and black pepper, place them on preheated grill over medium-high heat and cook for 8 minutes, flipping skewers from time to time.

5. Divide the skewers between plates and serve.

Nutritional value/serving: calories 260, fat 11,7, fiber 3, carbs 8,3, protein 31,7

Orange Salmon Bites

Preparation time: 10 minutes

Cooking time: 15 minutes

Servings: 4

Ingredients:

- 1 pound wild salmon, skinless, boneless and cubed
- 2 Meyer lemons, sliced
- ¼ cup balsamic vinegar
- ¼ cup orange juice
- A pinch of pink salt
- Black pepper to taste

Directions:

1. Heat up a small saucepan with the vinegar over medium heat, add the orange juice, stir, bring to a simmer for 1 minute and take off the heat.

2. Skewer salmon cubes and lemon slices, season with salt and black pepper, brush them with half of the vinegar mix, place on preheated grill over medium heat, cook for 4 minutes on each side.

3. Brush skewers with the rest of the vinegar mix, grill for 1 minute more, divide between plates and serve.

Nutritional value/serving: calories 290, fat 12,6, fiber 3, carbs 11,8, protein 40,3

Sushi Tuna Mix

Preparation time: 10 minutes

Cooking time: 5 minutes

Servings: 4

Ingredients:

- 1 small red onion, chopped
- ½ cup cilantro, chopped
- 1/3 cup olive oil+ 2 tablespoons
- 1 jalapeno pepper, chopped
- 2 tablespoons basil, chopped
- 3 tablespoons vinegar
- 3 garlic cloves, minced
- 1 teaspoon red pepper flakes
- 1 teaspoon thyme, chopped
- A pinch of sea salt
- Black pepper to taste
- 1 pound sushi grade tuna

- 2 avocados, pitted, peeled and chopped

- 6 ounces arugula

Directions:

1. In a bowl, mix 1/3 cup oil with onion, jalapeno, cilantro, basil, vinegar, garlic, parsley, pepper flakes, thyme, a pinch of salt and black pepper and whisk well.

2. Heat up a pan with the rest of the oil over medium-high heat, add tuna, season salt and black pepper, cook for 2 minutes on each side, transfer to a cutting board, leave aside to cool down and slice.

3. In a bowl, mix arugula with half of the chimichurri sauce you've made earlier, toss to coat well and divide between plates.

4. Also divide tuna slices, and avocado pieces and drizzle the rest of the sauce on top.

Nutritional value/serving: calories 938, fat 62,8, fiber 10, carbs 51,9, protein 43,8

Chili Salmon

Preparation time: 10 minutes

Cooking time: 15 minutes

Servings: 12

Ingredients:

- 1 and ¼ cups coconut, shredded

- 1 pound salmon meat, cubed

- 1/3 cup coconut flour

- A pinch of sea salt

- Black pepper to taste

- 1 egg

- 2 tablespoons coconut oil

- ¼ cup water

- 4 red chilies, chopped

- 3 garlic cloves, minced

- ¼ cup balsamic vinegar

- ½ cup honey

Directions:

1. In a bowl, mix coconut flour with a pinch of salt and stir.

2. In another bowl, whisk the egg with black pepper.

3. Put coconut in a third bowl.

4. Dip salmon cubes in flour, egg and coconut and place them all on a working surface.

5. Heat up a pan with the oil over medium-high heat, add salmon cubes, fry them for 3 minutes on each side, transfer them to paper towels, drain grease and divide them between plates.

6. Heat up a pan with the water over medium-high heat.

7. Add chilies, cloves, vinegar, honey and agar agar, stir well, bring to a gentle boil and simmer until all ingredients combine.

8. Drizzle this over salmon cubes and serve.

Nutritional value/serving: calories 180, fat 8,5, fiber 0,9, carbs 19,7, protein 7,7

Clams and Apple Mix

Preparation time: 10 minutes

Cooking time: 12 minutes

Servings: 2

Ingredients:

- 3 tablespoons ghee, melted

- 2 pound little clams, scrubbed

- 1 shallot, minced

- 2 garlic cloves, minced

- 1 cup cider

- 1 apple, cored and chopped

- Juice of ½ lemon

Directions:

1. Heat up a pan with the ghee over medium-high heat, add the shallot and garlic, stir and cook for 3 minutes.

2. Add cider, stir well and cook for 1 minute.

3. Add clams and thyme, cover and simmer for 5 minutes.

4. Add apple and lemon juice, stir, divide everything into bowls and serve.

Nutritional value/serving: calories 610, fat 23,6, fiber 2,9, carbs 43,7, protein 55,1

Paleo Vegetables Recipes

Lemon Spinach Mix

Servings: 2

Preparation time: 10 minutes

Cooking time: 15 minutes

Ingredients:

- 6 mushrooms, chopped

- A handful cherry tomatoes, cut in halves

- 3 handfuls spinach, torn

- 1 teaspoon ghee

- 2 tablespoons extra virgin olive oil

- 1 small red onion, sliced

- ½ teaspoon lemon rind, diced

- 1 garlic clove, minced

- A pinch of sea salt

- Black pepper to taste

- A pinch of nutmeg

- A drizzle of lemon juice

Directions:

1. Heat up a pan with the ghee over medium-high heat, add mushrooms, stir, cook for 4 minutes and transfer them to a plate.

2. Heat up the same pan with the olive oil over medium-high heat, add onion, stir and cook for 3 minutes.

3. Add tomatoes, a pinch of sea salt, pepper, lemon rind, nutmeg, and garlic, stir and cook for 3 minutes more.

4. Add spinach, stir and cook for 2-3 minutes.

5. Add lemon juice at the end, stir gently, transfer to plates and serve with mushrooms on top.

Nutritional value: calories 178, fat 16,5, carbs 9,9, fiber 2,3, protein 3,3

Nutmeg Celery Bake

Servings: 8

Preparation time: 10 minutes

Cooking time: 20 minutes

Ingredients:

- 1 white onion, finely chopped
- 1 celery head, chopped
- 2 and ½ tablespoons ghee
- 1 and ½ tablespoons coconut flour
- ½ teaspoon nutmeg
- A pinch of sea salt
- Black pepper to taste
- 1 and ½ cups coconut milk
- 2 tablespoons extra virgin olive oil
- ½ cup flax meal

Directions:

1. Heat up a pan with 1 tablespoon olive oil over medium-high heat, add celery, stir and cook for a few minutes until it browns a bit.

2. Add a pinch of sea salt and pepper, stir and transfer to a baking dish.

3. Heat up the same pan with the rest of the olive oil over medium heat, add onions, stir and cook for 4 minutes.

4. Add 1 and ½ tablespoons ghee, stir well and cook for 1-2 minutes.

5. Add the coconut flour, stir well for a few minutes and take off heat.

6. Add coconut milk, pepper to the taste and nutmeg and stir very well.

7. Return to medium heat and stir for 2 minutes more.

8. Add the rest of the ghee and flax meal, stir, pour everything over celery, toss to coat, place in the oven at 350 degrees F and bake for 15 minutes.

9. Divide between plates and serve.

Nutritional value/serving: calories 216, fat 20,6, carbs 8, fiber 4,6, protein 3,2

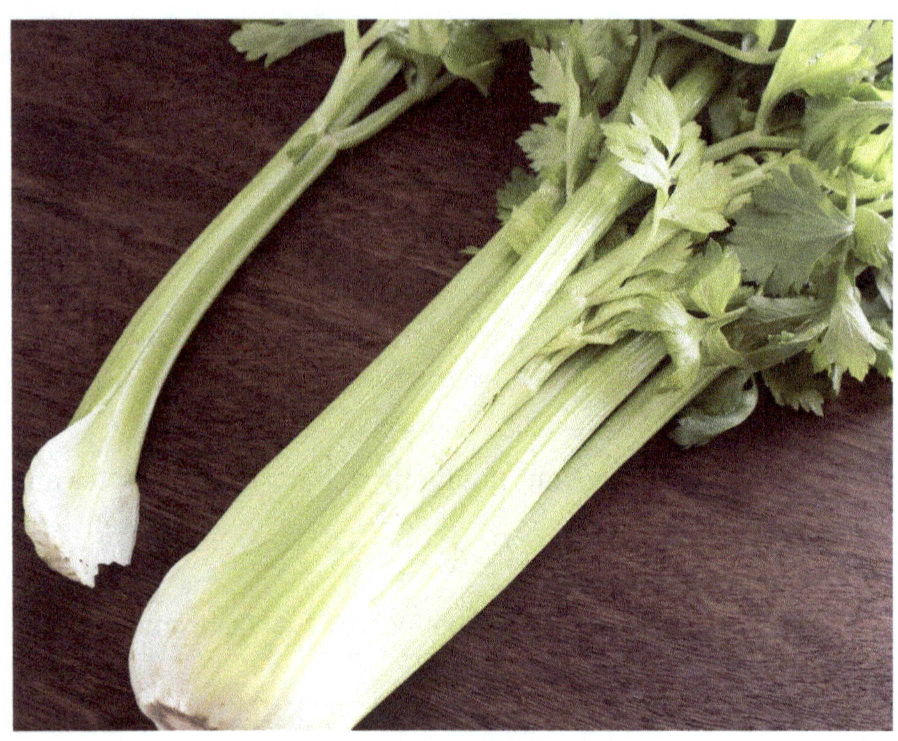

Rutabaga Pasta

Preparation time: 10 minutes

Cooking time: 25 minutes

Servings: 4

Ingredients:

For the sauce:

- 1 tablespoon shallot, chopped

- 1 garlic clove, minced

- ¾ cup cashews, soaked for a couple of hours and drained

- 2 tablespoons nutritional yeast

- ½ cup veggie stock

- A pinch of sea salt

- Black pepper to taste

- 2 teaspoons lemon juice

For the pasta:

- 1 cup cherry tomatoes, halved

- 5 teaspoons olive oil

- ¼ teaspoon garlic powder

- 2 rutabagas, peeled and cut into thin noodles

Directions:

1. Place tomatoes and rutabaga noodles on a lined baking sheet, drizzle the oil over them, season with a pinch of sea salt, black pepper and garlic powder, toss to coat, place in the oven at 400 degrees F and bake for 20 minutes.

2. Meanwhile, in a food processor, mix garlic with shallots, cashews, veggie stock, nutritional yeast, lemon juice, a pinch of sea salt and black pepper to taste and blend well.

3. Divide rutabaga pasta between plates, top with tomatoes and drizzle the sauce over them.

Nutritional value/serving: calories 298, fat 18,8, fiber 7,5, carbs 29,2, protein 9,1

Thyme Baked Tomatoes

Preparation time: 10 minutes

Cooking time: 50 minutes

Servings: 4

Ingredients:

- 4 garlic cloves, crushed
- 1 pound mixed cherry tomatoes
- 3 thyme springs, chopped
- A pinch of sea salt
- Black pepper to taste
- ¼ cup olive oil

Directions:

1. In a baking dish, mix tomatoes with a pinch of sea salt, black pepper, olive oil and thyme, toss to coat, place in the oven at 325 degrees F and bake for 50 minutes.

2. Divide tomatoes and pan juices between plates and serve.

Nutritional value/serving: calories 138, fat 13, fiber 2, carbs 6,6, protein 2

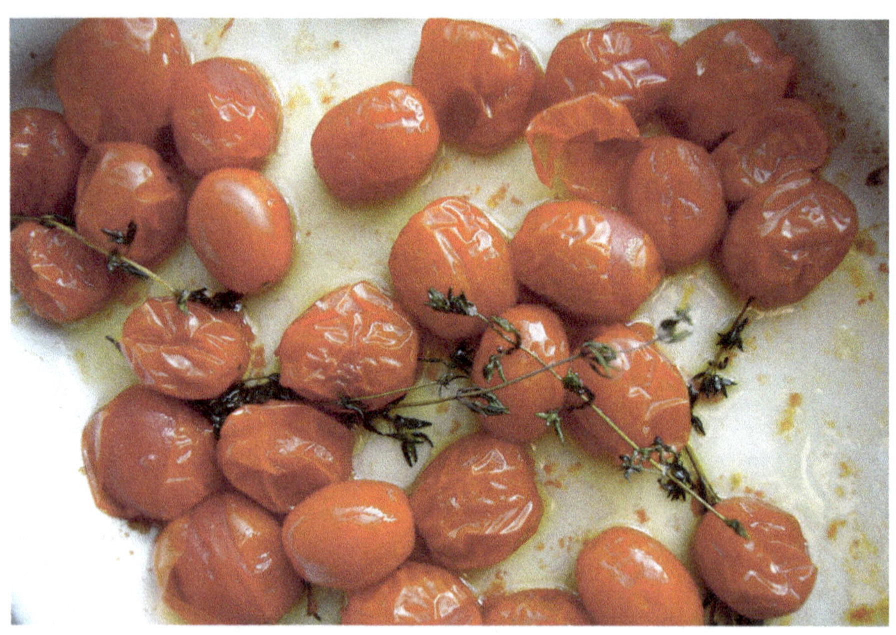

Tomato Bake

Preparation time: 10 minutes

Cooking time: 20 minutes

Servings: 2

Ingredients:

- 1 bunch basil, chopped

- 4 eggs

- 1 garlic clove, minced

- A pinch of sea salt

- Black pepper to taste

- ½ cup cherry tomatoes, halved

- ¼ cup almond cheese

Directions:

1. In a bowl, mix eggs with a pinch of sea salt, black pepper, almond cheese and basil and whisk well.

2. Pour this into a baking dish, arrange tomatoes on top, place in the oven at 350 degrees F and bake for 20 minutes.

3. Leave quiche to cool down, slice and serve.

Nutritional value/serving: calories 137, fat 8,9, fiber 0,6, carbs 5,5, protein 13,7

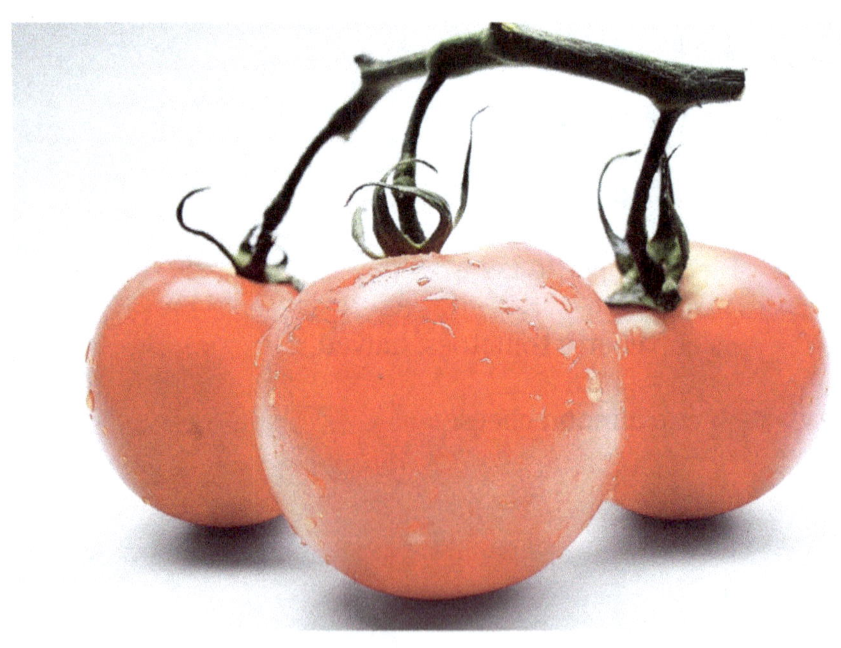

Tomato and Cucumber Mix

Preparation time: 30 minutes

Cooking time: 4 minutes

Servings: 4

Ingredients:

- 1 teaspoon coconut sugar

- 3 cups cherry tomatoes, halved

- ¼ teaspoon cumin, ground

- 1 tablespoon sherry vinegar

- A pinch of sea salt

- 1 red onion, chopped

- 2 cucumbers, sliced

- ¼ cup olive oil

- Black pepper to taste

Directions:

1. Put cherry tomatoes in a bowl, season with coconut sugar, a pinch of salt and black pepper and leave aside for 30 minutes.

2. Drain tomatoes and pour juices into a pan.

3. Heat this up over medium heat, add cumin and vinegar and bring to a simmer.

4. Cook for 4 minutes, take off heat and mix with olive oil.

5. Add tomatoes, onion and cucumber to this mix, toss well, divide between plates and serve.

Nutritional value/serving: calories 171, fat 13,1, fiber 3, carbs 14,4, protein 2,5

Paleo Salad Recipes

Pork and Lettuce Salad

Servings: 4

Preparation time: 10 minutes

Cooking time: 5 minutes

Ingredients:

- 2 lettuce heads, torn

- 2 cups pork, already cooked and shredded

- 1 avocado, pitted, peeled and chopped

- 1 cup cherry tomatoes, cut in halves

- 1 green bell pepper, sliced

- 2 green onions, thinly sliced

- A pinch of sea salt

- Black pepper to taste

- Juice of ½ lime

- 1 tablespoon apple cider vinegar

- ¼ cup BBQ sauce

- 2 tablespoons extra virgin olive oil

Directions:

1. In a small bowl, mix oil with lime juice, vinegar, black pepper and BBQ sauce and whisk well.

2. Heat up a pan over medium heat, add pork meat and heat it up.

3. Meanwhile, in a salad bowl, mix lettuce leaves with tomatoes, bell pepper, avocado and green onions.

4. Add pork, drizzle the BBQ dressing, toss to coat and serve.

Nutritional value/serving: calories 349, fat 20,2, carbs 19,9, fiber 5,7, protein 24,3

Shrimp and Crab Salad

Servings: 6

Preparation time: 3 hours

Cooking time: 0 minutes

Ingredients:

- 8 ounces, baby shrimp, already cooked, peeled, deveined and chopped
- 8 ounces crab meat, already cooked
- 2/3 cup homemade mayonnaise
- 2/3 cup yellow onion, chopped
- 2/3 cup celery, chopped
- 2 tablespoons Dijon mustard
- Black pepper to taste
- ¼ teaspoon onion powder
- ½ teaspoon garlic powder
- 1 tablespoon hot sauce

Directions:

1. In a salad bowl, mix shrimp with crab meat, onion, and celery.

2. In another bowl, mix mayo with mustard, pepper, onion powder, garlic powder and hot sauce and stir well.

3. Pour this over seafood salad, toss to coat and keep in the fridge for 3 hours before you serve it.

Nutritional value/serving: calories 198, fat 9,9, carbs 9, fiber 0,6, protein 16,8

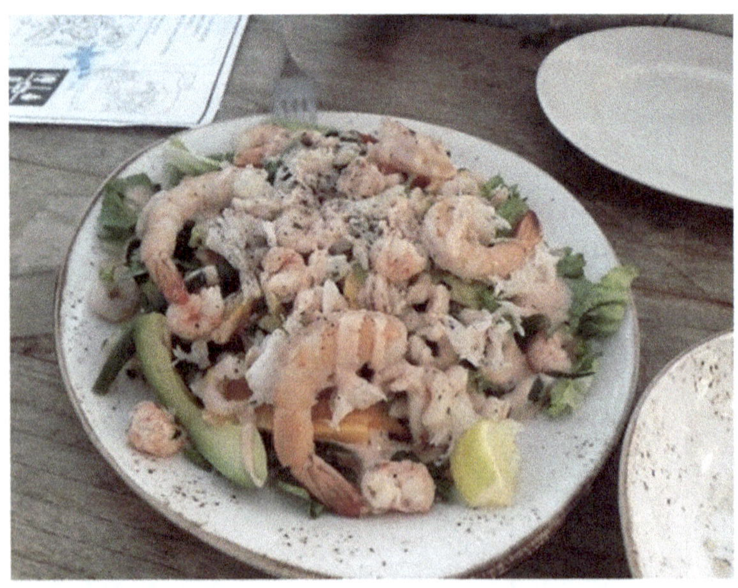

Cilantro Beef Salad

Preparation time: 10 minutes

Cooking time: 15 minutes

Servings: 4

Ingredients:

- 1 tablespoon chili powder
- 1 teaspoon onion powder
- ½ teaspoon garlic powder
- 1 teaspoon cumin, ground
- 2 teaspoons paprika
- 3 tablespoons olive oil
- A pinch of cayenne pepper
- 1 pound beef, ground
- 3 cups cilantro, chopped
- Juice from 1 lime
- A pinch of sea salt
- Black pepper to taste

- 1 romaine lettuce head, chopped

- 1 avocado, pitted, peeled and chopped

- 1 small red onion, chopped

- Some black olives, pitted and chopped

- 1 red bell pepper, chopped

- ½ cup Pico de gallo

Directions:

1. In a bowl, mix chili powder with paprika, onion and garlic powder, ½ teaspoon cumin, cayenne and some black pepper and stir.

2. Heat up a pan with 1 tablespoon oil over medium heat, add beef, stir and cook for 7 minutes.

3. Add spice mix, stir and cook until meat is done.

4. Meanwhile, in your food processor, blend 1 cup cilantro with lime juice, ½ teaspoon cumin, a pinch of salt, black pepper to taste and 2 tablespoons oil and pulse well.

5. In a salad bowl, mix lettuce leaves with avocado, 2 cups cilantro, onion, bell pepper, olives and Pico de gallo and stir.

6. Divide this between plates, top with beef and drizzle the salad dressing on top.

Nutritional value/serving: calories 464, fat 29,4, fiber 6,2, carbs 15,8, protein 27,1

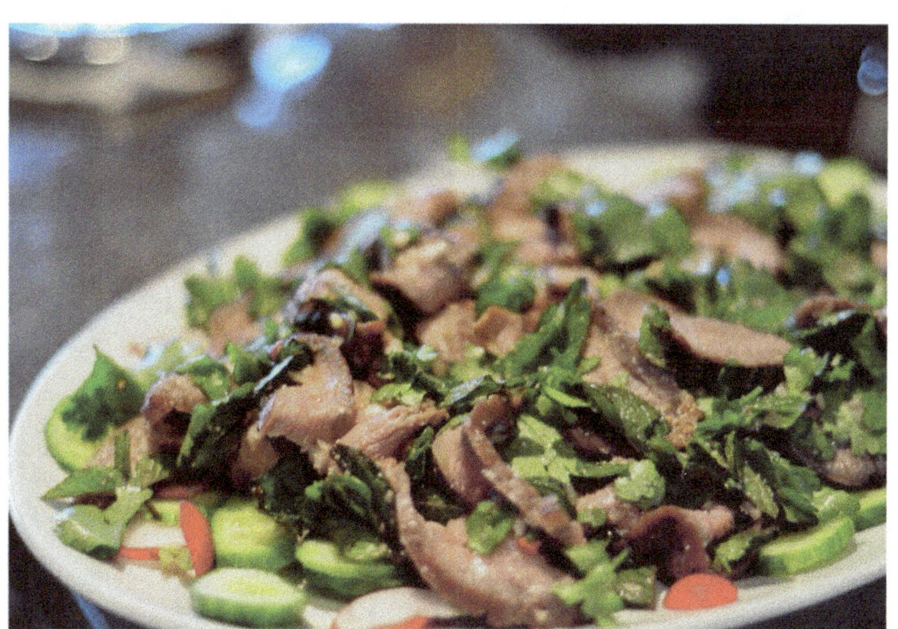

Lemon Berries and Honeydew Salad

Preparation time: 10 minutes

Cooking time: 0 minutes

Servings: 6

Ingredients:

- 1 cup blackberries, halved
- 2 cups honeydew, sliced
- 8 ounces prosciutto
- 3 tablespoons chives, chopped
- Juice of 1 lemon
- Zest from 1 lemon
- 1 shallot, chopped
- 2 cup cantaloupe, sliced
- A pinch of sea salt
- Black pepper to taste

Directions:

1. In a large salad bowl, mix blackberries with prosciutto, honeydew, cantaloupe, chives, lemon juice and zest, shallot, a pinch of sea salt and black pepper to taste, toss to coat and serve cold.

Nutritional value/serving: calories 107, fat 2,4, fiber 2,3, carbs 13,3, protein 9,1

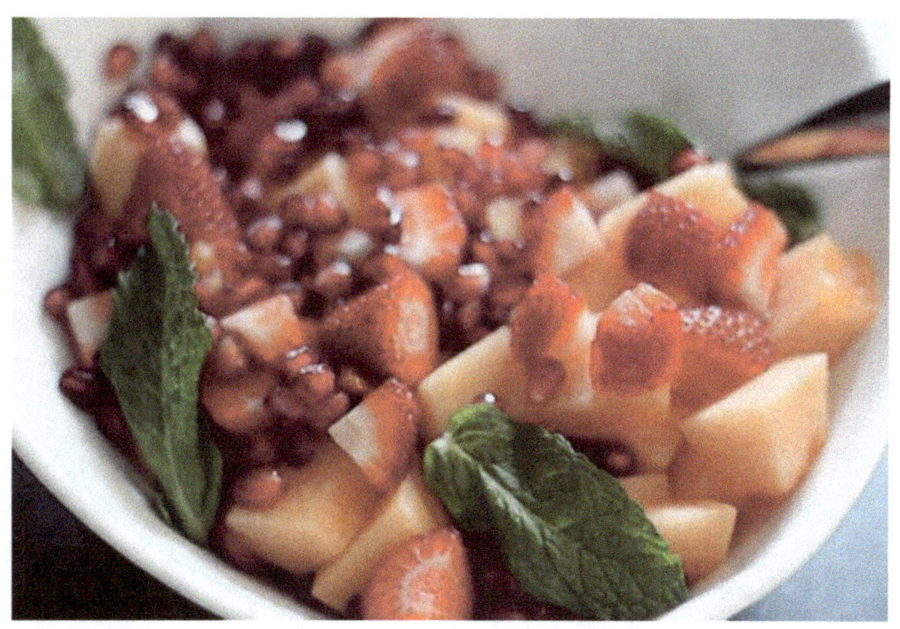

Brussels Sprouts and Pecan Salad

Preparation time: 10 minutes

Cooking time: 7 minutes

Servings: 2

Ingredients:

- 1 red onion, chopped

- 12 Brussels sprouts, sliced

- A pinch of sea salt

- Black pepper to taste

- 1 tablespoon olive oil

- 1/3 cup pecans, chopped

- ¼ cup raisins

- 2/3 cup hemp seeds

- ½ red apple, cored and chopped

Directions:

1. Heat up a pan with the oil over medium heat, add onion, stir and cook for a few minutes.

2. Add Brussels sprouts, cook for 4 minutes, take off
    heat and leave aside to cool down.

3. Add apple pieces, hemp seeds, raisins, a pinch of sea
    salt, black pepper and pecans, stir salad and serve.

Nutritional value/serving: calories 522, fat 34,8, fiber 10,2, carbs 42,1, protein 19,2

Lime Kale and Lettuce Salad

Preparation time: 10 minutes

Cooking time: 0 minutes

Servings: 1

Ingredients:

- 1 carrot, grated
- A handful kale, chopped
- 1 small lettuce head, chopped
- 1 tablespoon tahini paste
- 1 tablespoon olive oil
- A pinch of sea salt
- Black pepper to taste
- Juice of ½ lime
- A pinch of garlic powder

Directions:

1. In a salad bowl, mix carrots with kale and lettuce leaves.

2. In a blender, mix tahini with a pinch of salt, black pepper, garlic powder, lime juice and oil and pulse well.

3. Pour this over salad, toss to coat well and serve.

Nutritional value/serving: calories 264, fat 22,2, fiber 3,8, carbs 16,9, protein 4,2

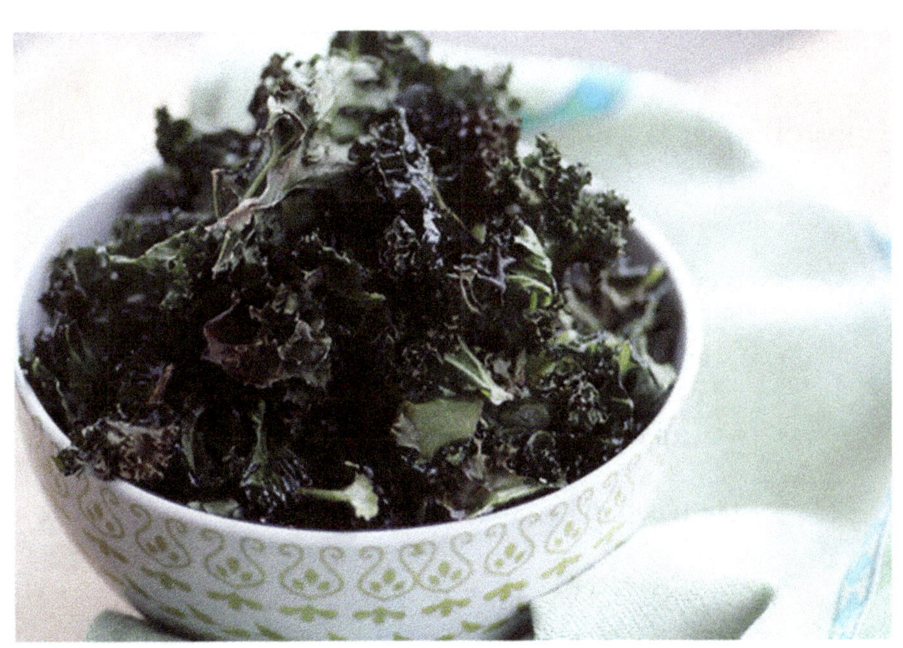

Paleo Dessert Recipes

Maple Cobbler

Preparation time: 10 minutes

Cooking time: 30 minutes

Servings: 5

Ingredients:

- ¾ cup maple syrup
- 6 cups strawberries, halved
- 1 tablespoon lemon juice
- ½ cup coconut flour
- 1/4 teaspoon baking soda
- ½ cup water
- 3 and ½ tablespoons coconut oil
- A drizzle of avocado oil

Directions:

1. Grease a baking dish with a drizzle of avocado oil and leave aside.
2. In a bowl, mix strawberries with maple syrup, sprinkle some flour and add lemon juice.
3. Stir very well and pour into baking dish.
4. In another bowl, mix flour with baking soda and stir well.
5. Add coconut and mix until the whole thing crumbles in your hands.
6. Add ½ cup water and spread over strawberries.
7. Place in the oven at 375 degrees F and bake for 30 minutes.
8. Take cobbler out of the oven, leave aside for 10 minutes and then serve.

Nutritional value/serving: calories 318, fat 11,2, fiber 9,5, carbs 55, protein 3,2

Cocoa Almond Bowls

Preparation time: 3 hours

Cooking time: 0 minutes

Servings: 4

Ingredients:

- 1 cup almond milk
- 2 avocados, peeled and pitted
- ¾ cup cocoa powder
- 1 teaspoon vanilla extract
- ¾ cup maple syrup
- ¼ teaspoon cinnamon
- Walnuts chopped for serving

Directions:

1. Put avocados in a kitchen blender and pulse well.

2. Add cocoa powder, almond milk, maple syrup, cinnamon and vanilla extract and pulse well again.

3. Pour into serving bowls, top with walnuts and keep in
    the fridge for 2-3 hours before you serve it.

Nutritional value/serving: calories 536, fat 36,1, fiber 12,9,

carbs 60,7, protein 6,2

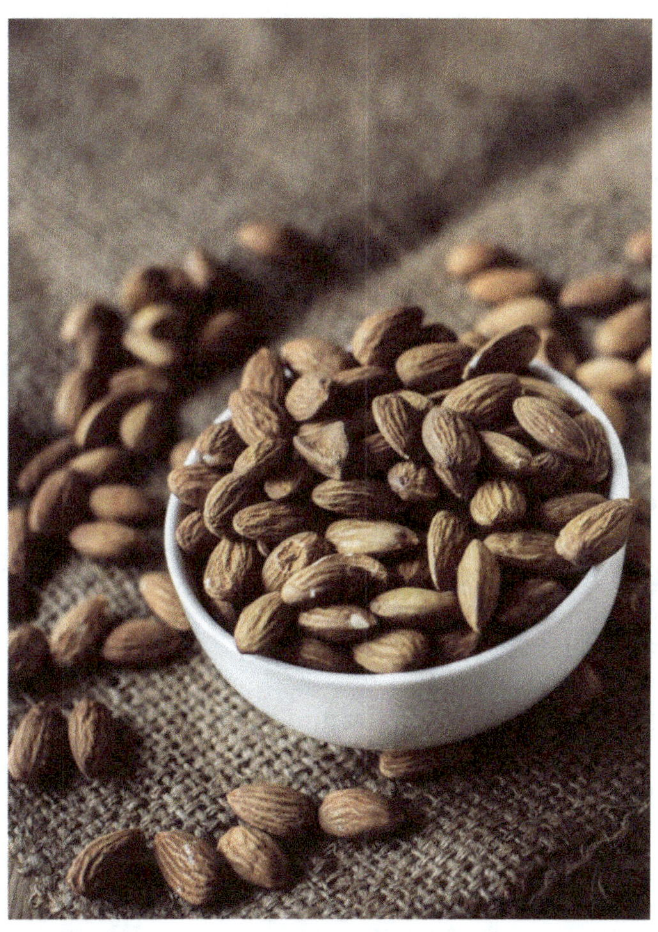

Dates and Plums Smoothie Bowls

Preparation time: 2 hours

Cooking time: 0 minutes

Servings: 4

Ingredients:

- 1 cup dates, pitted and chopped
- 3 cups plums, chopped
- 2 and ½ cups water
- 1 teaspoon lemon juice

Directions:

1. Put dates and plums in a food processor and blend well.
2. Add water gradually and pulse a few more times.
3. Add lemon juice, pulse for a few more seconds, transfer to a bowl and keep in the freezer for 2 hours.
4. Scoop into dessert cups and serve right away!

Nutritional value/serving: calories 148, fat 0,3, carbs 39,4,

fiber 4,3, protein 1,5

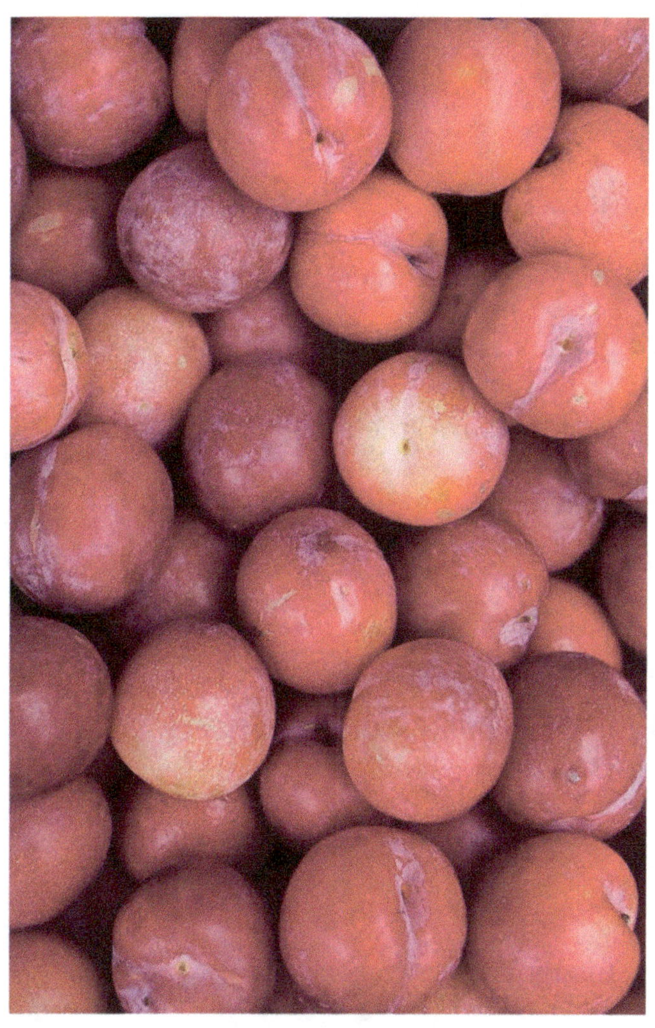

Green Avocado Bowls

Preparation time: 6 minutes

Cooking time: 0 minutes

Servings: 4

Ingredients:

- ½ cup coconut water

- 1 and ½ cup avocado, chopped

- 2 tablespoons green tea powder

- 2 teaspoons lime zest

- 1 tablespoon honey

- Melted coconut butter for serving

- 1 mango thinly sliced for serving

Directions:

1. In a blender, mix water with avocado, green tea powder and lime zest and pulse well.

2. Add honey and pulse again well.

3. Transfer to a bowl, top with coconut butter spread all over and serve with sliced mango.

Nutritional value/serving: calories 216, fat 15,7, fiber 8,6, carbs 18,4, protein 4,7

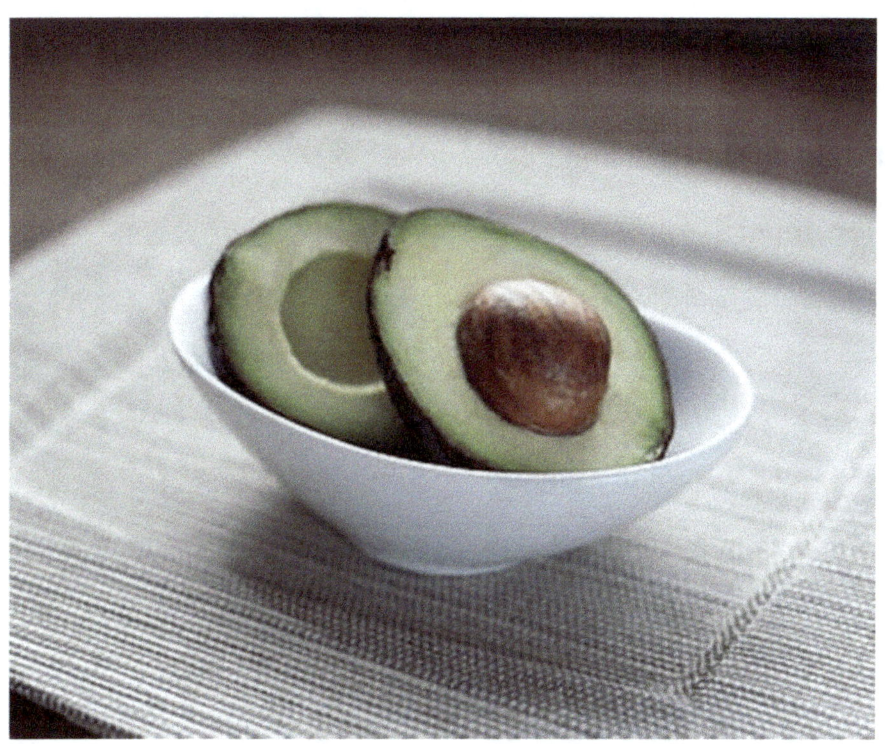

Paleo Snacks and Appetizer Recipes

Thyme Zucchini Fries

Preparation time: 10 minutes

Cooking time: 12 minutes

Servings: 4

Ingredients:

- 1 zucchini, thinly sliced
- A pinch of sea salt
- Black pepper to taste
- 1 teaspoon thyme, dried
- 1 egg
- 1 teaspoon garlic powder
- 1 cup almond flour

Directions:

1. In a bowl, whisk the egg with a pinch of salt.

2. Put the flour in another bowl and mix it with thyme, black pepper, and garlic powder.

3. Dredge zucchini slices in the egg mix and then in flour.

4. Arrange chips on a lined baking sheet, place in the oven at 450 degrees F and bake for 6 minutes on each side,

5. Serve the zucchini chips as a snack.

Nutritional value/serving: calories 106, fat 8,2, fiber 2,1, carbs 5,2, protein 5,1

Cheese Bites

Preparation time: 5 minutes

Cooking time: 10 minutes

Servings: 24 pieces

Ingredients:

- 1/3 cup tomatoes, chopped
- ½ cup bell peppers, mixed and chopped
- ½ cup tomato sauce
- 4 ounces almond cheese, cubed
- 2 tablespoons basil, chopped
- Black pepper to taste

Directions:

1. Divide tomato and bell pepper pieces into a muffin tray.

2. Also divide the tomato sauce, basil and almond cheese cubes, sprinkle black pepper at the end, place

cups in the oven at 400 degrees F and bake for 10 minutes.

3. Arrange the meal on a platter and serve.

Nutritional value/serving: calories 59, fat 4,5, fiber 0,1, carbs 2, protein 2,5

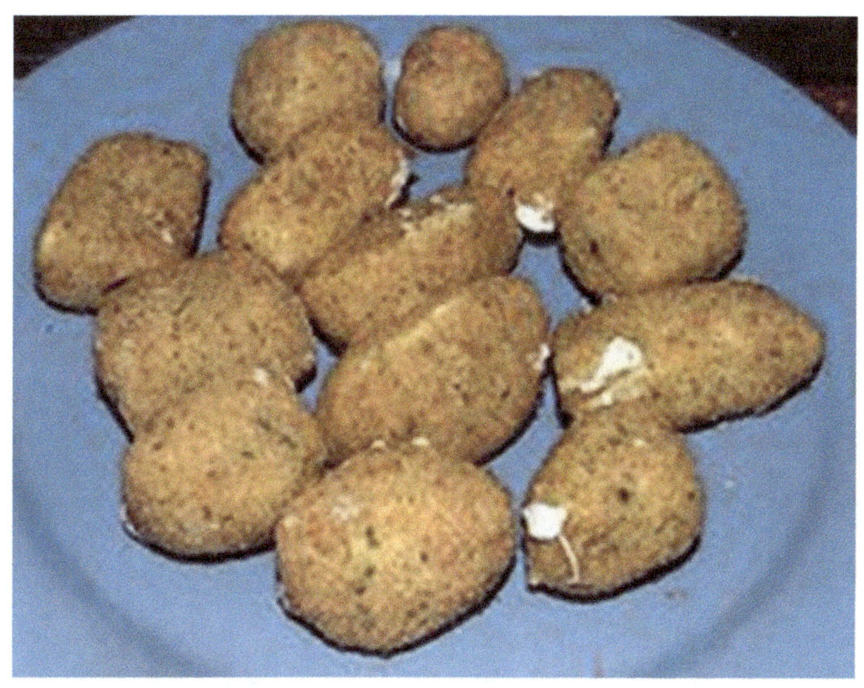

Turkey Balls

Preparation time: 10 minutes

Cooking time: 40 minutes

Servings: 20

Ingredients:

- 1 pound turkey meat, ground
- 1 tablespoon coconut oil, melted
- 1 yellow onion, chopped
- 1 egg
- 1 cup coconut flour
- 1 teaspoon Italian seasoning
- A pinch of sea salt
- Black pepper to taste
- 2 tablespoons parsley, chopped

Directions:

1. In a bowl, mix turkey meat with half of the flour, a pinch of salt, black pepper, Italian seasoning, parsley,

onion, egg and hot sauce and stir well.

2. Put the rest of the flour in another bowl.

3. Shape 20 turkey meatballs and dip each one in flour.

4. Heat up a pan with the oil over medium-high heat,
    add meatballs, cook them for 4 minutes on each side,
    transfer to paper towels to remove any excess grease,
    place all of them on a platter and serve.

Nutritional value/serving: calories 71, fat 2,6, fiber 2,2,
carbs 4,1, protein 7,7

Coconut Chicken Bites

Preparation time: 10 minutes

Cooking time: 20 minutes

Servings: 4

Ingredients:

- 1 pound chicken tenders
- 1 egg, whisked
- A pinch of sea salt
- 1/3 cup coconut, unsweetened and shredded
- ¼ cup coconut flour

Directions:

1. In a bowl, mix coconut with coconut flour and a pinch of sea salt and stir.
2. Put whisked egg in another bowl.

3. Dip chicken pieces in egg, then in coconut mixture, arrange them all on a lined baking sheet and bake at 350 degrees F for 25 minutes.

4. Serve as a snack.

Nutritional value/serving: calories 330, fat 13,6, fiber 8,1, carbs 13,6, protein 36,9

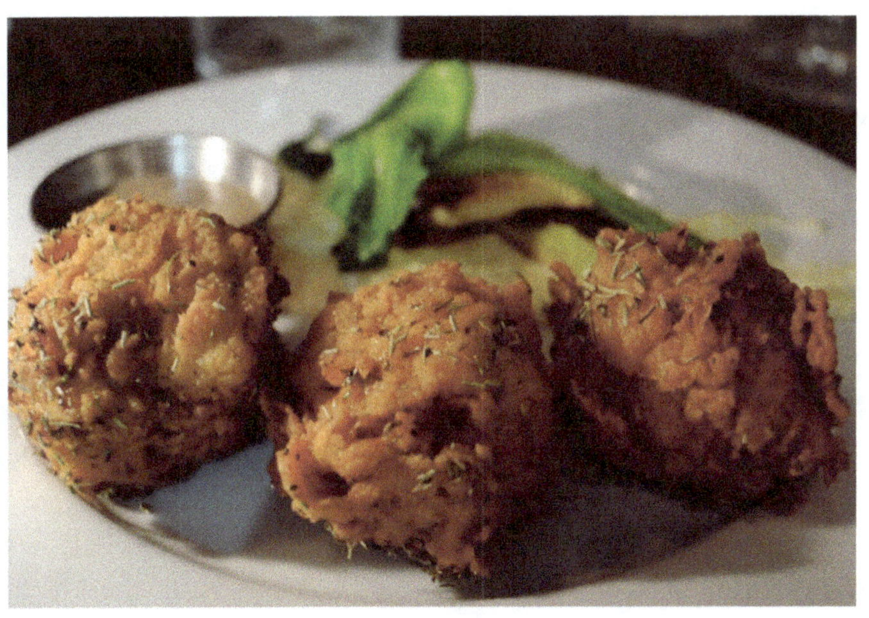

Paleo Recipes for Breakfast

Avocado and Pumpkin Sandwich

Servings: 2

Preparation time: 10 minutes

Cooking time: 10 minutes

Ingredients:

- 4 ounces pumpkin flesh, peeled

- 4 slices paleo coconut bread

- 1 avocado, pitted and peeled

- 1 carrot, grated

- 2 lettuce leaves

Directions:

1. Spread the pumpkin flesh in a tray, bake at 350 degrees F for 10 minutes, transfer to a bowl and mash it with a fork.

2. Put the avocado in separate bowl and mash it with a fork.

3. Spread avocado on 2 paleo bread slices, also divide the grated carrot, mashed pumpkin and the lettuce leaves on each and top them with the other 2 bread slices and serve for breakfast.

Nutritional value/serving: calories 310, fat 21,7, fiber 20,1, carbs 26,6, protein 12,6

Turkey and Cranberry Sandwich

Servings: 1

Preparation time: 5 minutes

Cooking time: 0

Ingredients:

- 2 turkey breast slices, skinless, boneless and roasted
- 2 tablespoons walnuts, toasted and chopped
- 2 slices paleo coconut bread
- 2 tablespoons cranberry chutney
- ¼ cup baby arugula

Directions:

1. In a bowl, mix the walnuts with the chutney, stir and spread on one paleo slice of bread.
2. Add the turkey slices and the arugula, top with the other slice of bread and serve.

Nutritional value/serving: calories 347, fat 12,7, fiber 13,6, carbs 37,4, protein 28,6

Coconut Berry Smoothie

Servings: 2

Preparation time: 5 minutes

Cooking time: 0

Ingredients:

- 2 cups blueberries

- 1 teaspoon lemon zest, grated

- ½ cup coconut milk

- 1 teaspoon cinnamon powder

- 3 cups water

Directions:

1. In a blender, combine all the ingredients, pulse well, divide into 2 glasses and serve for breakfast.

Nutritional value/serving: calories 222, fat 14,8, fiber 4,9, carbs 24,5, protein 2,5

Lemon Kale Smoothie

Serving: 2

Preparation time: 5 minutes

Cooking time: 0

Ingredients:

- 1 small cucumber, peeled and chopped

- 1 green apple, chopped

- Juice of ½ lemon

- Juice of ½ lime

- 1 tablespoon ginger, finely grated

- 1 cup kale, chopped

- 1 cup coconut water

Directions:

1. In a blender, combine all the ingredients, pulse well, divide into 2 glasses and serve for breakfast.

Nutritional value/serving: calories 138, fat 1, fiber 5,8, carbs 32,1, protein 3,6

Cabbage and Berry Smoothie

Servings: 2

Preparation time: 5 minutes

Cooking time: 0

Ingredients:

- 1 small red bell pepper, seeded and roughly chopped

- 5 strawberries, halved

- 1 tomato, cut into 4 wedges

- 1 cup red cabbage, chopped

- ½ cup raspberries

- 8 ounces water

- 2 ice cubes for serving

Directions:

1. In a blender, combine all the ingredients and pulse well. Divide into glasses and serve.

Nutritional value: calories 200, fat 5, fiber 11, carbs 20, protein 9

Mint Berry Smoothie

Servings: 2

Preparation time: 10 minutes

Cooking time: 0

Ingredients:

- 1 and ½ cups kiwi, chopped

- 1 and ½ cups frozen strawberries, chopped

- 8 mint leaves

- 2 cups crushed ice

- ¼ cup water

Directions:

1. In a blender, combine all the ingredients and pulse well. Divide into glasses and serve.

Nutritional value/serving: calories 59, fat 0,5, fiber 4,7, carbs 13,7, protein 1,9

Paleo Soup and Stew Recipes

Lemon Turkey and Zucchini Stew

Servings: 3

Preparation time: 10 minutes

Cooking time: 30 minutes

Ingredients:

- 1 yellow onion, chopped

- 1 tablespoon coconut oil, melted

- 15 ounces turkey meat, cooked, thinly sliced

- 1 red bell pepper, chopped

- 1 carrot, thinly sliced

- 1 celery stick, chopped

- 1 tomato, chopped

- 2 garlic cloves, minced

- 2 cups chicken stock

- 1 tablespoon lemon juice

- Black pepper to the taste

- 1 zucchini, chopped

- A handful parsley leaves, chopped

Directions:

1. Heat up a pan with the oil over medium-high heat, add turkey, onion, celery and carrot, stir and cook for 3 minutes.

2. Add red bell pepper, tomatoes and garlic, stir and cook 1 minute.

3. Add lemon juice, stock and pepper, stir, bring to a boil, cover pan, reduce heat to medium and cook for 10 minutes.

4. Add zucchini, stir, cook for 12 more minutes, divide into bowls, sprinkle the parsley on top and serve.

Nutritional value/serving: calories 345, fat 12,4, fiber 3,3, carbs 13,5, protein 44,3

Beef and Greens Stew

Servings: 4

Preparation time: 10 minutes

Cooking time: 5 hours

Ingredients:

- 6 plantains, skinless and cubed
- 2 pounds beef meat, cubed
- 3 cups collard greens, chopped
- A pinch of sea salt and black pepper
- 3 cups water
- ½ cup sweet paprika
- 3 tablespoons allspice
- ¼ cup garlic powder
- 1 teaspoon chili powder
- 1 teaspoon cayenne pepper

Directions:

1. In a slow cooker, mix all the ingredients, toss, cover and cook on High for 5 hours.

2. Divide into bowls and serve.

Nutritional value/serving: calories 827, fat 19,6, fiber 14,2, carbs 104,5, protein 19,9

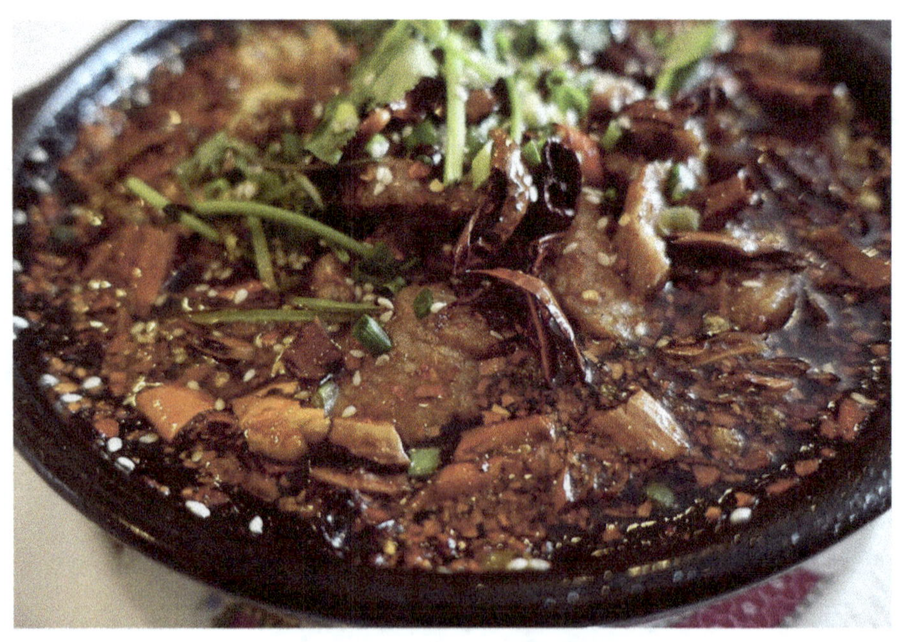

Pumpkin and Chicken Stew

Servings: 6

Preparation time: 15 minutes

Cooking time: 8 hours

Ingredients:

- 5 garlic cloves, minced

- 2 celery stalks, chopped

- 2 yellow onions, chopped

- 2 carrots, chopped

- 30 ounces homemade pumpkin puree

- 2 quarts chicken stock

- 2 cups chicken breast, skinless, boneless and cubed

- ¼ cup coconut flour

- Black pepper to taste

- ½ pound baby spinach

- ¼ teaspoon cayenne pepper

Directions:

1. In a slow cooker, combine all the ingredients except the spinach, cover and cook on Low for 7 hours and 50 minutes.

2. Add the spinach, cook on Low for 10 more minutes, divide into bowls and serve.

Nutritional value/serving: calories 222, fat 3,6, fiber 10,8, carbs 30, protein 18,6

Masala Lamb Stew

Servings: 4

Preparation time: 15 minutes

Cooking time: 1 hour and 50 minutes

Ingredients:

- 1 and ½ pounds lamb meat, cubed

- 1 tablespoon coconut oil, melted

- ½ red chili, seedless and chopped

- 1 brown onion, chopped

- 3 garlic cloves, minced

- 2 celery sticks, chopped

- 2 and ½ teaspoons garam masala powder

- 1 teaspoon fennel seeds

- A pinch of sea salt and black pepper

- 1 and ¼ teaspoons turmeric powder

- 1 and ½ teaspoons ghee, melted

- 14 ounces coconut milk

- 1 cup water

- 1 tablespoon lemon juice

- 2 carrots, chopped

- A handful parsley leaves, finely chopped

Directions:

1. Heat up a pan with the oil over medium-high heat, add the lamb, stir and brown for 4 minutes.

2. Add celery, chili and onion, stir and cook 1 minute more.

3. Reduce heat to medium, add garam masala, garlic, ghee, fennel, and turmeric, stir and cook 1 minute.

4. Add salt, pepper, tomato paste, coconut milk and water, stir, bring to a boil, reduce heat to low, cover and cook for 1 hour.

5. Add carrots and cook for 40 minutes more, stirring occasionally.

6. Add lemon juice and parsley, stir, transfer to bowls and serve.

Nutritional value/serving: calories 829, fat 54, fiber 9,5, carbs 38,7, protein 45,1

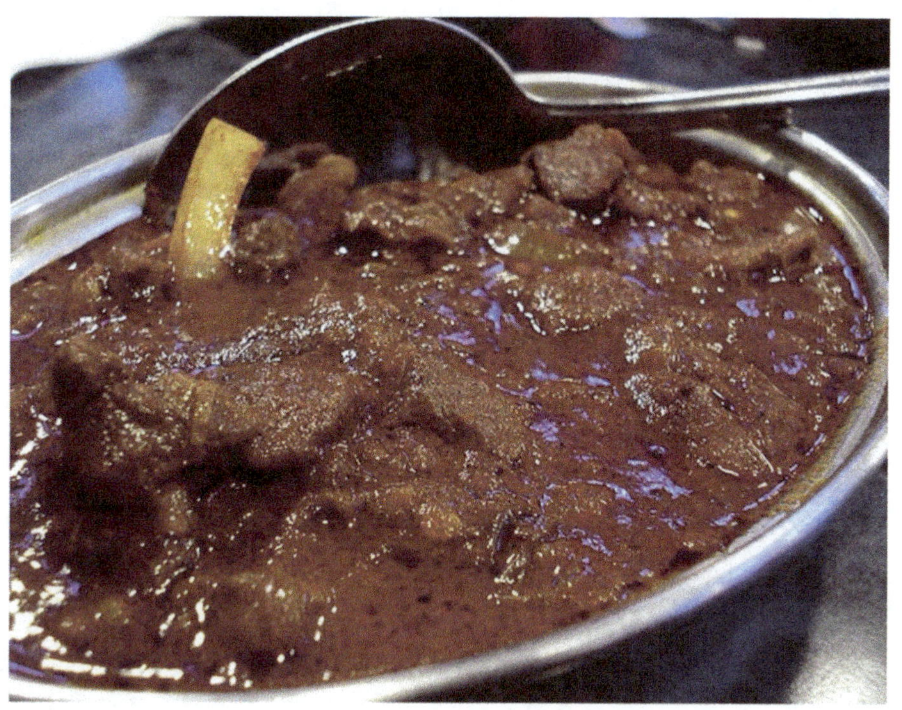

Root Veggie Stew

Servings: 6

Preparation time: 10 minutes

Cooking time: 1 hour and 10 minutes

Ingredients:

- 4 pounds mixed root vegetables (parsnips, carrots, rutabagas, beets, celery root, turnips), chopped
- 6 tablespoons extra virgin olive oil
- 1 garlic head, cloves separated and peeled
- ½ cup yellow onion, chopped
- Black pepper to taste
- 25 ounces fresh tomatoes, peeled, chopped
- 1 tablespoon tomato paste
- 2 cups kale leaves, torn
- 1 teaspoon oregano, dried

Directions:

1. In a baking dish, mix all root vegetables with black pepper, half of the oil and garlic, toss to coat, and bake at 450 degrees F for 45 minutes.

2. Heat up a pot with the rest of the oil over medium-high heat, add onions and sauté for 2-3 minutes

3. Add tomato paste, tomatoes, salt, pepper and the oregano, stir, bring to a simmer, reduce heat to low and cook for 10 minutes.

4. Add baked veggies and kale, toss, cook for 5 more minutes, divide into bowls and serve.

Nutritional value/serving: calories 293, fat 19,2, fiber 9,8, carbs 32,7, protein 2,2

Herbed Chicken and Olives Stew

Servings: 4

Preparation time: 15 minutes

Cooking time: 2 hours

Ingredients:

- 10 garlic cloves, peeled

- 30 black olives, pitted

- 2 pounds chicken breasts, skinless, boneless and cubed

- 2 cups chicken stock

- 25 ounces tomatoes, peeled, chopped

- 2 tablespoon rosemary, chopped

- 2 tablespoons parsley, chopped

- 2 tablespoons basil, chopped

- A pinch of sea salt and black pepper

- A drizzle of extra virgin olive oil

Directions:

1. Heat up a large saucepan with a drizzle of olive oil over medium-high heat, add the chicken, salt and pepper, and cook for 4 minutes.

2. Add garlic, stir and brown for 2 minutes more.

3. Add chicken stock, tomatoes, olives, thyme, and rosemary, stir, cover saucepan and bake in the oven at 325 degrees F for 1 hour.

4. Add parsley and basil, stir, bake for 45 more minutes, divide into bowls and serve.

Nutritional value/serving: calories 553, fat 24,8, fiber 4,1, carbs 13, protein 68,5

Paleo Side Dish Recipes

Garlic and Basil Tomatoes

Servings: 4

Preparation time: 5 minutes

Cooking time: 20 minutes

Ingredients:

- 2 tablespoons extra virgin olive oil
- 20 ounces colored cherry tomatoes, halved
- 6 garlic cloves, finely minced
- A pinch of sea salt and black pepper
- 1 tablespoon basil leaves, finely chopped

Directions:

1. In a baking dish, combine all the ingredients, place in the oven at 375 degrees F and bake for 20 minutes.

2. Divide between plates and serve as a side dish.

Nutritional value/serving: calories 91, fat 7,4, fiber 1,9, carbs 6,8, protein 2,1

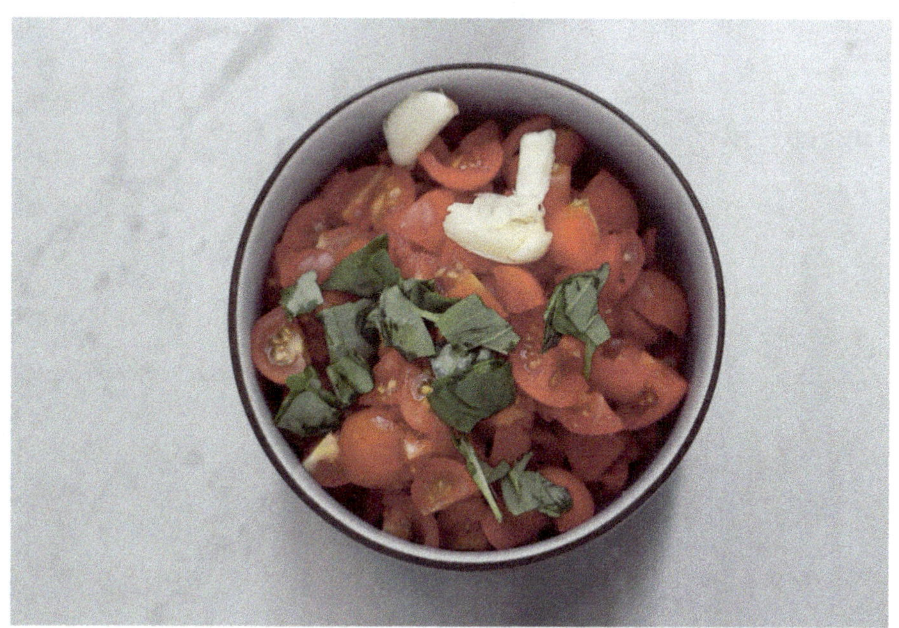

Garlic Spinach

Servings: 3

Preparation time: 10 minutes

Cooking time: 33 minutes

Ingredients:

- 3 cups spinach, torn
- 3 yellow onions, sliced
- 3 garlic cloves, finely minced
- A pinch of sea salt and black pepper
- 10 mushrooms, sliced
- 1 tablespoon coconut oil, melted
- 1 tablespoon balsamic vinegar
- 1 tablespoon ghee

Directions:

1. Heat up a pan with the oil and ghee over medium-high heat, add garlic and onions, stir and cook for 10 minutes.

2. Reduce temperature to low and cook onions for 20 minutes, stirring from time to time.

3. Add vinegar, mushrooms, salt and pepper, stir and cook for 10 minutes.

4. Add spinach, stir, cook for 3 minutes more, take off heat, divide between plates and serve as a side dish.

Nutritional value: calories 146, fat 9,2, fiber 3,7, carbs 14,4, protein 4,2

Parsley Carrot Mash

Servings: 4

Preparation time: 6 minutes

Cooking time: 20 minutes

Ingredients:

- 1 pound rutabaga, peeled and chopped
- A pinch of sea salt and black pepper
- 4 tablespoons ghee
- 1 pound carrots, chopped
- 1 tablespoon parsley, chopped

Directions:

1. Put rutabaga and carrots in a pot, add water to cover, place on stove, bring to a boil over medium heat and cook for 20 minutes.

2. Drain carrots and rutabaga, transfer them to a bowl, mash with a potato masher, mix with ghee, salt and

pepper, stir well, divide between plates, sprinkle parsley on top and serve as a side dish.

Nutritional value/serving: calories 200, fat 13, fiber 5,7, carbs 12,4, protein 2,4

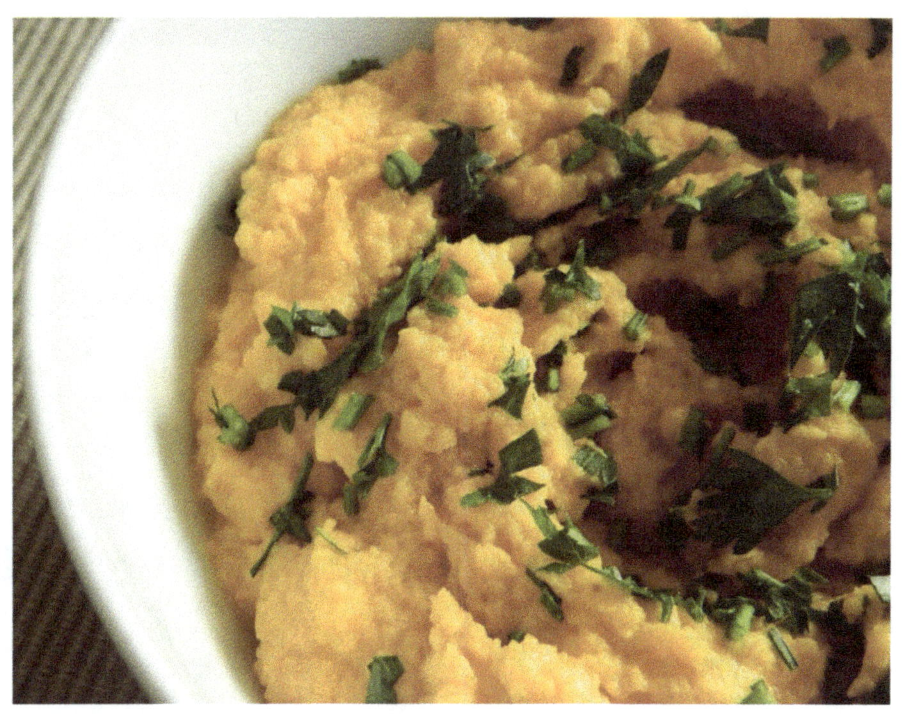

Balsamic Peppers and Capers Mix

Servings: 4

Preparation time: 10 minutes

Cooking time: 1 hour

Ingredients:

- 6 bell peppers (green, yellow and red)

- 1 garlic clove, finely minced

- 2 tablespoon capers

- 2 tablespoons extra virgin olive oil

- ¼ cup balsamic vinegar

- A pinch of sea salt and black pepper

- 2 tablespoons parsley, finely chopped

Directions:

1. Arrange bell peppers on a lined baking sheet, place them in the oven at 400 degrees F and bake for 40 minutes.

2. Transfer bell peppers to a bowl, cover and leave them aside for 10 minutes.

3. Peel the peppers, discard seeds, cut into strips and transfer them to a bowl.

4. Add sea salt and pepper, vinegar, oil, garlic, capers and parsley, toss to coat, divide between plates and serve as a side dish.

Nutritional value/serving: calories 123, fat 7,5, fiber 2,6, carbs 14,2, protein 2

Herbed Potatoes

Servings: 3

Preparation time: 10 minutes

Cooking time: 25 minutes

Ingredients:

- 2 pounds sweet potatoes, cut into wedges
- A pinch of sea salt and black pepper
- ¼ cup ghee, melted
- 3 teaspoons thyme and rosemary, dried

Directions:

1. In a bowl, mix potato wedges with ghee, salt, pepper and dried herbs and toss to coat.
2. Spread potatoes on a lined baking sheet and bake in the oven at 425 degrees F for 25 minutes.
3. Divide between plates and serve as a side dish.

Nutritional value: calories 512, fat 7,7, fiber 13,1, carbs 85,6, protein 4,9

Lemon Chili Cabbage

Servings: 4

Preparation time: 10 minutes

Cooking time: 30 minutes

Ingredients:

- 1 green cabbage head, cut into medium wedges
- A pinch of sea salt and black pepper
- A pinch of red chili flakes
- A pinch of garlic powder
- 2 tablespoons extra virgin olive oil
- Juice of 2 lemons

Directions:

1. Brush the cabbage with olive oil, salt and pepper, sprinkle garlic powder and pepper flakes, arrange it on a lined baking sheet and bake at 450 degrees F for 30 minutes, flipping the cabbage wedges halfway.

2. Divide between plates, drizzle the lemon juice on top
    and serve.

Nutritional value: calories 118, fat 7,3, fiber 4,8, carbs 14,
protein 2,7

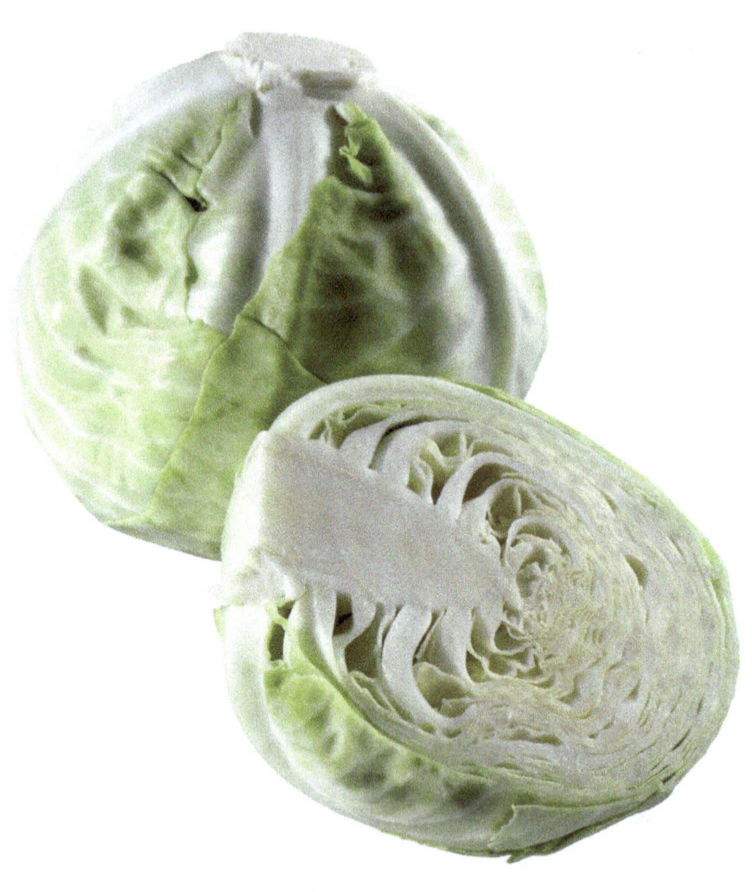

Paleo Meat Recipes

Pork and Berry Mix

Servings: 4

Preparation time: 10 minutes

Cooking time: 30 minutes

Ingredients:

- 1 cup blueberries
- ½ teaspoon thyme, dried
- 2 pounds pork loin
- 1 tablespoon balsamic vinegar
- ½ teaspoon red chili flakes
- 1 teaspoon ginger powder
- A pinch of sea salt
- Black pepper to taste
- 2 tablespoon water

Directions:

1. Put pork loin in a baking dish and season with a pinch of sea salt and pepper to taste.

2. Heat up a pan over medium heat, add blueberries and mix with vinegar, water, thyme, chili flakes and ginger.

3. Stir well, cook for 5 minutes and pour over pork loin.

4. Place in the oven at 375 degrees F and bake for 25 minutes.

5. Take pork out of the oven, leave aside for 5 minutes, slice, divide between plates and serve with blueberries sauce.

Nutritional value/serving: calories 572, fat 31,7, carbs 5,4, fiber 0,9, protein 62,3

Salsa Pork Mix

Servings: 4

Preparation time: 12 hours and 10 minutes

Cooking time: 8 hours and 20 minutes

Ingredients:

- ½ cup paleo salsa

- ½ cup beef stock

- ½ cup enchilada sauce

- 3 pounds organic pork shoulder

- 2 green chilies, chopped

- 1 tablespoon garlic powder

- 1 tablespoon chili powder

- 1 teaspoon onion powder

- 1 teaspoon cumin, ground

- 1 teaspoon sweet paprika

- Black pepper to taste

Directions:

1. In a bowl, mix chili powder with onion and garlic one.

2. Add cumin, paprika and pepper to taste and stir everything.

3. Add pork, rub well and keep in the fridge for 12 hours.

4. Transfer pork to a slow cooker, add enchilada sauce, stock, salsa and green chilies, stir, cover and cook on Low for 8 hours.

5. Transfer pork to a plate, leave aside to cool down and shred.

6. Strain sauce from slow cooker into a pan, bring to a boil over medium heat and simmer for 8 minutes stirring all the time.

7. Add shredded pork to the sauce, stir, reduce heat to medium and cook for 20 more minutes.

8. Divide between plates and serve hot.

Nutritional value: calories 1013, fat 73, carbs 4,3, fiber 1,6, protein 80,4

Smoked Pork Ribs

Servings: 4

Preparation time: 15 minutes

Cooking time: 2 hours and 47 minutes

Ingredients:

- 1 tablespoon smoked paprika

- ½ tablespoon onion powder

- ½ tablespoon garlic powder

- ½ teaspoon cayenne pepper

- 4 pounds baby ribs

- 1 cup paleo BBQ sauce

- 4 teaspoons Sriracha

- ¼ cup cilantro, chopped

- ¼ cup chives, chopped

- ¼ cup parsley, chopped

- Black pepper to taste

Directions:

1. In a bowl, mix paprika with onion powder, garlic powder, pepper and cayenne and stir well.

2. Add ribs, toss to coat and arrange them on a lined baking sheet.

3. Place in the oven at 325 degrees F and bake them for 2 hours and 30 minutes.

4. In a bowl, mix BBQ sauce with Sriracha and stir well.

5. Take ribs out of the oven, mix them with BBQ sauce, place them on preheated grill over medium-high heat and cook for 7 minutes on each side.

6. Divide ribs between plates, sprinkle chives, cilantro, and parsley on top and serve.

Nutritional value/serving: calories 1483, fat 122,3, fiber 1,1, carbs 9,5, protein 81,8

Sage Pork

Servings: 4

Preparation time: 10 minutes

Cooking time: 30 minutes

Ingredients:

- 8 sage springs

- 4 pork chops, bone-in

- 4 tablespoons ghee

- 4 garlic cloves, crushed

- 1 tablespoon coconut oil

- A pinch of sea salt

- Black pepper to taste

Directions:

1. Season pork chops with a pinch of sea salt and pepper to taste.

2. Heat up a pan with the oil over medium high heat, add pork chops and cook for 10 minutes turning them often.

3. Take pork chops off heat, add ghee, sage, and garlic and toss to coat.

4. Return to heat, cook for 4 minutes often stirring, divide between plates and serve.

Nutritional value/serving: calories 402, fat 36, fiber 0,1, carbs 1, protein 18,2

Balsamic Pork Mix

Servings: 4

Preparation time: 10 minutes

Cooking time: 45 minutes

Ingredients:

- 1 yellow onion, chopped

- 1 organic pork tenderloin

- 2 pears, chopped

- 2 garlic cloves, minced

- 1 tablespoon chives, chopped

- ¼ cup walnuts, chopped

- 3 tablespoons balsamic vinegar

- Black pepper to taste

- ½ cup chicken stock

- 1 tablespoon coconut oil

- 1 tablespoon lemon juice

Directions:

1. In a bowl, mix walnuts with pear, chives, pepper and lemon juice and stir well.

2. Heat up a pan with the oil over medium-high heat, add tenderloin and brown for 3 minutes on each side.

3. Reduce heat, add onion and garlic, stir and cook for 2 minutes.

4. Add balsamic vinegar, stock, pear mix, stir, place in the oven at 400 degrees F and bake for 20 minutes.

5. Take pork out of the oven, leave aside for 4 minutes, slice, divide between plates and serve with pear salsa on top.

Nutritional value/serving: calories 271, fat 11,2, fiber 4,4, carbs 20,1, protein 24,6

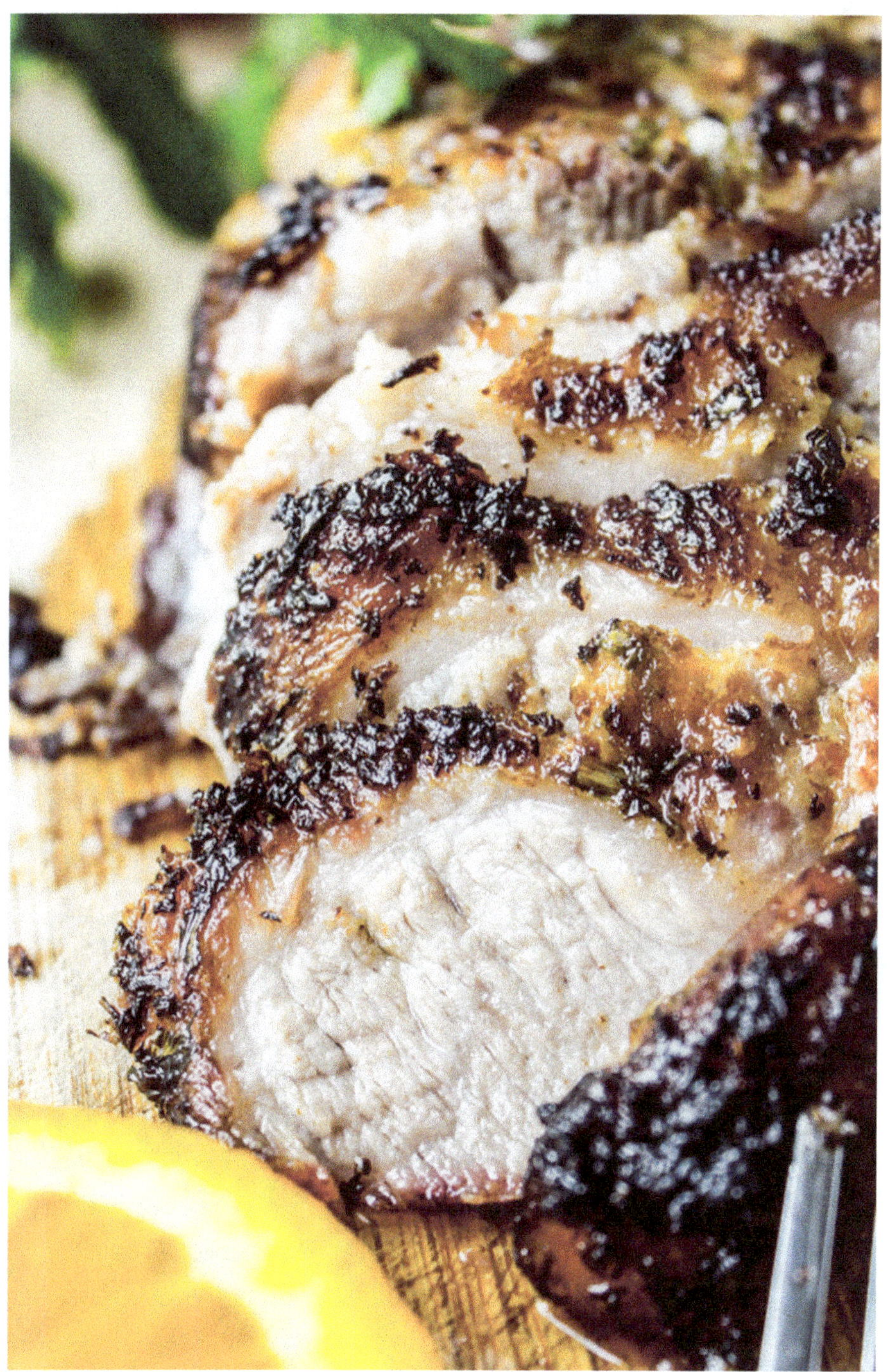

Pork with Carrots and Sauce

Servings: 4

Preparation time: 10 minutes

Cooking time: 45 minutes

Ingredients:

- 15 oz turkey mince
- A handful arugula
- Black pepper to taste
- 1 grass fed pork tenderloin
- 1 tablespoon coconut oil

For the puree:

- 1 sweet potato, chopped
- 3 carrots, chopped
- A pinch of sea salt
- Black pepper to taste
- 1 tablespoon curry paste

For the sauce:

- 2 tablespoons balsamic vinegar

- 1 teaspoon mustard

- 2 shallots, chopped

- Black pepper to taste

- 4 tablespoons extra virgin olive oil

Directions:

1. Slice pork tenderloin in half horizontally but not all the way and open it up.

2. Use a meat tenderizer to even it up.

3. Place turkey mince in the middle, roll pork around it, tie with twine, season pepper to taste and leave to one side.

4. Heat up an oven proof pan with the coconut oil over medium-high heat, add pork roll, cook for 3 minutes on each side, place in the oven at 350 degrees F and bake for 25 minutes.

5. Meanwhile, put potatoes and carrots in a large saucepan, add water to cover, bring to a boil over

medium-high heat, cook for 20 minutes, drain and transfer to a food processor.

6. Pulse a few times until you obtain a puree, add a pinch of sea salt and pepper to taste, blend again, transfer to a bowl and leave aside.

7. Take pork roll out of the oven, slice and divide between plates.

8. Heat up a pan with the olive oil over medium-high heat, add shallots, stir and cook for 10 minutes.

9. Add balsamic vinegar, mustard, pepper, stir well and take off heat. Divide carrots puree next to pork slices, drizzle vinegar sauce on to and serve with arugula on the side.

Nutritional value/serving: calories 495, fat 29,5, carbs 2,2, fiber 17,5, protein 21,8

www.ingramcontent.com/pod-product-compliance
Lightning Source LLC
Chambersburg PA
CBHW071447030726
47593CB00003B/934